COVID-19 AND LIVABLE CITIES IN ASIA AND THE PACIFIC

GUIDANCE NOTE

DECEMBER 2020

ASIAN DEVELOPMENT BANK

ADB

Contents

Tables and Figures

Tables

Figures

Acknowledgments

COVID-19 and Livable Cities in the Asia and Pacific Guidance Note is part of a series of sector guidance notes by Asian Development Bank (ADB) in response to COVID-19, directed by Robert Guild and Woochong Um of ADB's Sustainable Development and Climate Change Department (SDCC). This *Livable Cities* guidance note was prepared by the Urban Sector Group of the Sustainable Development and Climate Change Department (SDCC), Asian Development Bank (ADB). The Urban Sector Group is composed of Hong Soo Lee, senior urban specialist; Virinder Sharma, senior urban development specialist; Lara Arjan and Sunghoon Kris Moon, urban development specialists; Aldrin Plaza, urban development officer; Lindy Lois Gamolo, senior operations assistant; Elyn Ruth Ravancho, associate operations analyst; and Haezel Barber, Gabrielle Elga Reyes, and Karen Lapitan, consultants. Manoj Sharma, chief of the Urban Sector Group; and Robert Guild, chief sector officer of SDCC, supervised the preparation of this guidance note.

Key contributions were given by the Urban Sector Group Committee that comprised the Central and West Asia Urban Development and Water Division; East Asia Urban and Social Sectors Division; Pacific Urban Development, Water Supply and Sanitation Division; South Asia Urban Development and Water Division; Southeast Asia Urban Development and Water Division; Private Sector Operations Department; and the Office of Public-Private Partnership. The Urban Climate Change Resilience Trust Fund team and the Cities Development Initiative for Asia Trust Fund team also provided valuable inputs.

This guidance note and its recommended interventions seek to be of use to cities of ADB's developing member countries in crafting and implementing strategies, programs, and policy measures aimed at overcoming the consequences of the coronavirus disease (COVID-19) crisis and supporting recovery during and after the pandemic.

Abbreviations

ADB	Asian Development Bank
COVID-19	coronavirus disease
DMC	developing member country
ICT	information and communication technology
MSMEs	micro, small, and medium-sized enterprises
m^2	square meter
OP4	ADB Strategy 2030 Operational Plan for Priority 4: Making Cities More Livable
WASH	water, sanitation, and hygiene

Executive Summary

Declared on 11 March 2020 as a global pandemic by the World Health Organization (WHO), the coronavirus disease (COVID-19) has become the most urgent crisis today. It has affected the normal lives of citizens—disrupting their routines and causing them severe physical, social, and economic distress. In Asia and the Pacific, the poor and the vulnerable people in cities are the most adversely affected by this pandemic. While various diseases and epidemics have influenced the development of cities over the centuries, a pandemic like COVID-19 has caused an unprecedented global impact on cities across the world.

This *Livable Cities* guidance note aims to support cities in developing member countries (DMCs) of the Asian Development Bank (ADB). It seeks to effectively respond to the crisis in the immediate term, and to "build back better" in the short- and medium-term while continuously adapting to the "new normal" with respect to human behaviors, social interactions, and business practices. The note is anchored on the core principles outlined under *ADB Strategy 2030 Operational Plan for Priority 4: Making Cities More Livable* (OP4). The recommended interventions are aligned with the three major outcomes of OP4: (i) coverage, quality, efficiency, and reliability of services in urban areas improved; (ii) urban planning and financial sustainability of cities strengthened; and (iii) urban environment, climate resilience, and disaster management of cities improved.

In the immediate term, the proposed key approaches toward creating livable cities are to (i) remodel public spaces, commercial offices, industrial buildings, and civic institutions to adapt to COVID-19; (ii) ensure continued smooth operations of urban water and wastewater utilities; provide essential water, sanitation, and hygiene (WASH) services; and improve solid waste and medical waste management; (iii) address the special needs of informal settlements and vulnerable people; (iv) address the residents' changing travel needs during the pandemic; and (v) effectively use information and communication technology solutions. These immediate actions should be part of the short- and medium-term efforts.

The proposed actions in the short and medium-term are to (i) enhance inclusivity through greater social protection measures for the most vulnerable groups; (ii) improve urban services and infrastructure and effectively use technologies and digital solutions; (iii) revisit urban planning to strategically incorporate lessons from the pandemic; (iv) strengthen the financial sustainability of local governments and build capacities of urban institutions and other stakeholders; (v) focus on healthy and environmentally sustainable cities; and (vi) build resilient cities, enabling them to absorb shocks and stresses due to pandemics, disasters, and climate change.

This guidance note also takes into account the public health and economic impacts of the pandemic. In addition to livable cities, ADB's series of COVID-19 guidance notes cover other key sectors and thematic areas including education, energy, public-private partnerships, transport, and water.

ADB will align its urban sector portfolio to help DMCs address the impacts of COVID-19. ADB's Urban Sector Group has an average annual commitment of $2 billion, which can be used to design livable cities projects. These projects are envisioned to help cities in DMCs become more healthy, inclusive, and resilient. The projects will also support local economic development and create jobs for the citizens. The tragedy caused by the COVID-19 pandemic brings about lessons that DMCs can learn from as they transition into the "new normal." This health crisis also serves as an opportunity to reduce inequalities of access and make cities more safe, healthy, environmentally sustainable, resilient, and inclusive.

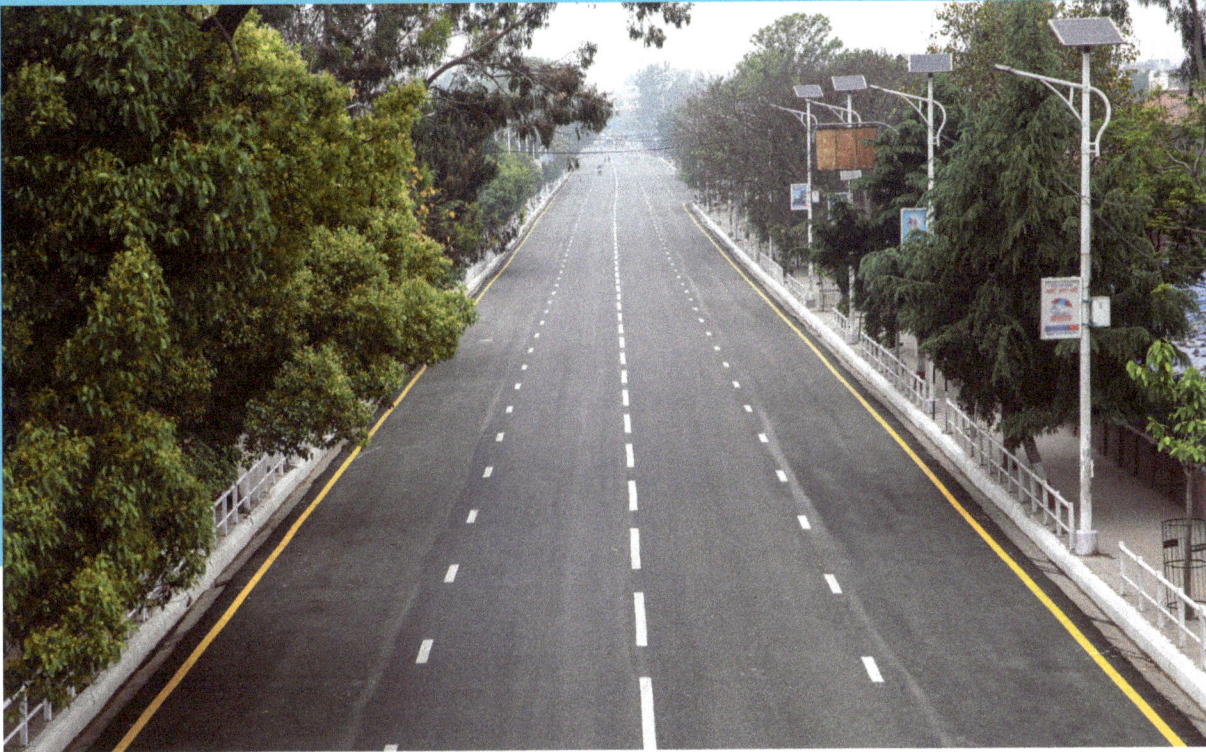

Cities fall silent. The COVID-19 pandemic has put cities to a standstill, which led to empty streets, closed establishments, and interrupted social services.

1 Introduction

Cities have been experiencing unprecedented urban issues and challenges that call for new attempts to respond from a different perspective. The changed working and living patterns—brought about by the inadequacy of essential urban services, jeopardized urban health, diminishing social inclusiveness, contracting urban economy and job security, weakening urban resilience, and the inevitable non-face-to-face system—require new ways of planning and operations at both the public and private sectors for the cities in developing member countries (DMCs) of the Asian Development Bank (ADB).

As urban planning has begun to secure public health and sanitation and to resolve environmental pollution problems, it is necessary to prepare a more comprehensive urban management structure not only for immediate actions but also for short- and medium-term measures on the premise that infectious diseases such as coronavirus disease (COVID-19) become indigenous.

In line with the core principles of ADB Strategy 2030 Operational Plan for Priority 4: Making Cities More Livable (OP4), this guidance note intends to support ADB and the cities in DMCs adopting to the "new normal" with respect to human behaviors, social interactions, and business practices.[1]

---

[1]   ADB. 2019. *Strategy 2030 Operational Plan for Priority 4: Making Cities More Livable, 2019–2024*. Manila.

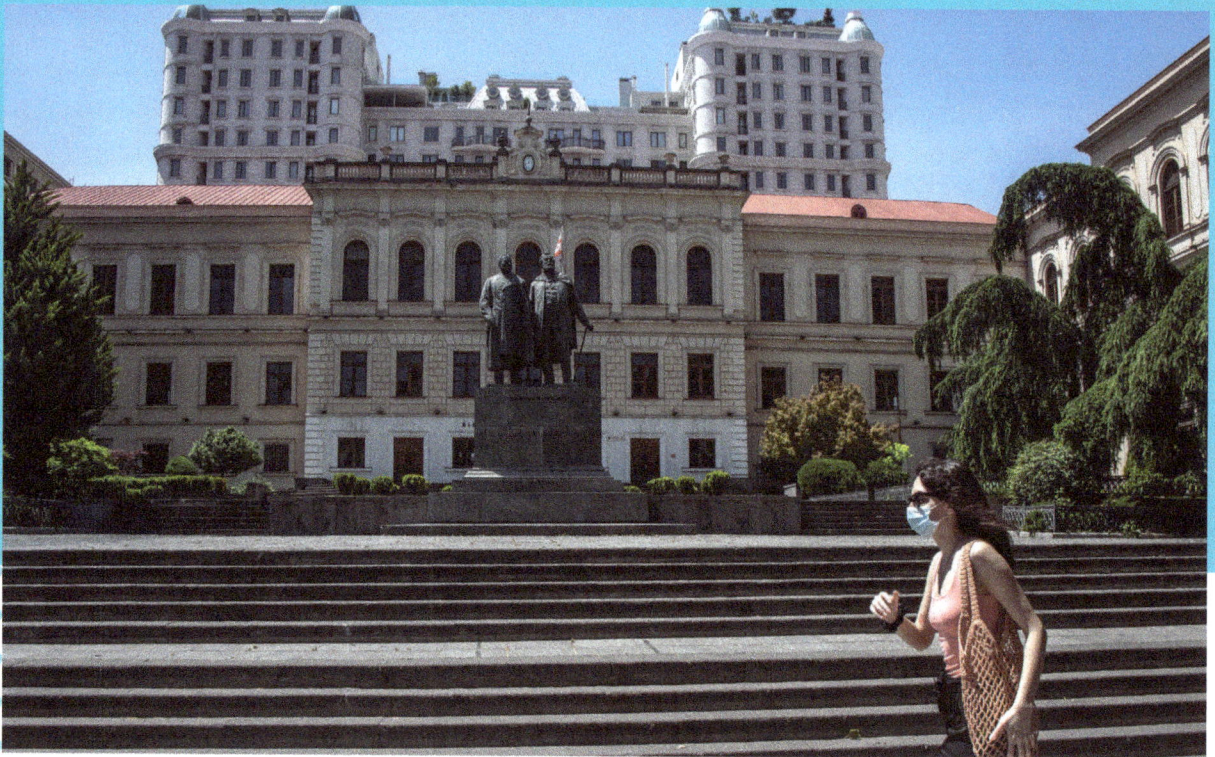

Urban economic crisis. The COVID-19 pandemic has pushed many establishments to close down, which would bring crisis at the macro and micro levels.

② Issues and Challenges

Cities in DMCs are facing challenges that have been further aggravated by COVID-19. Some of these are elaborated here.

Inadequate urban and social infrastructure. Most cities in DMCs face inadequate urban services and deficits in basic urban infrastructure (e.g., transport, water supply, sanitation and wastewater management, solid waste management, energy, and telecommunications) and social infrastructure (e.g., health care, education, public and community facilities, including affordable housing).[2] The inadequate urban services, which are a huge challenge before the COVID-19 pandemic, have placed outbreak-affected areas at a greater disadvantage due to disruptions in regular operations.

Intensified impacts on vulnerable population. The population of cities in DMCs with high-density environments, especially those in informal settlements and slums, are highly exposed to the risks of COVID-19. The impact of the crisis, which exacerbates existing inequalities, is highest among the urban poor, who experience the dual challenges of increased vulnerabilities to the disease and reduced opportunities of livelihoods due to economic restrictions. Living in overcrowded, unsafe, and unhealthy conditions, the vulnerable people (e.g., slum residents, pavement dwellers, squatters, homeless

---

[2]   The addition of 1.2 billion new residents in cities in Asia and the Pacific between 2019 and 2050 will have profound implications on the region's economy, society, and environment. See UNESCAP. 2019. *The Future of Asian and Pacific Cities*. Bangkok.

persons, informal sector workers, and migrant workers) find it difficult to comply with the prescribed social distancing measures. Their problems are aggravated by substandard housing and a lack of access to safe water, sanitation, and hygiene (WASH) facilities. There are also reports of increased gender-based violence and elevated stress due to living within small and confined spaces during the enforced stay-at-home period.[3] The inability to stock food supplies by residents in informal settlements and the closed street markets due to the quarantine restrictions further deteriorate the vulnerable people's living and health conditions.

Ineffective information and communication technology system. Despite the high penetration of internet and personal mobile phones in DMCs, cities often lack integrated systems and equal access to information and communication technology (ICT) that are required to effectively address a crisis of this magnitude. The incomplete and, sometimes, asymmetric information due to inadequate local ICT systems triggers and aggravates citizens' anxiety and engenders panic reactions, as seen in many cities in DMCs in the first few months of the pandemic. Irresponsible fake news and unsubstantiated messages through social media cause more harm as the ICT systems of several DMCs are not capable of countering such propaganda with factual and accurate information—which citizens need during a pandemic. The lack of reliable data from service providers that own and operate open source data makes it difficult for governments to complement their own datasets, which are a critical requirement to productive and effective functioning of comprehensive smart city platforms.

Urban economic crisis at the macro and micro levels. Cities, which contribute a substantial part of gross domestic product in DMCs, have not been able to sufficiently withstand the economic shocks of COVID-19. The severe hardships faced by micro, small, and medium-sized enterprises (MSMEs) is evident; and workers, especially those in low-income categories, find it difficult to secure work-from-home arrangements. Similarly, cities have felt the economic impacts of the pandemic due to, among others, reduced revenues of local governments (e.g., taxes, tariffs, and intergovernment transfers), irregular and reduced remittances from overseas workers, and disruptions in value chains and production networks across countries. Given the inadequate social protection systems, supporting MSMEs, workers, and the vulnerable people in cities has been a challenge. The existing political, economic, and regulatory systems in DMCs often limit the cities' systemic and holistic response to support workers and MSMEs and revitalize economies.

Strained local government planning and management. Local governments, which are at the forefront of tackling the crisis on the ground, are required to immediately respond to emergency situations which, at times, overwhelm their capacities in terms of resources, financing, personnel, and systems and logistics. Their performance in emergency preparedness, crisis management, and operational readiness has been put to the test to meet the demands of their national governments, regulatory systems, and numerous stakeholders.

---

[3] UN Women. 2020. *The First 100 Days of the COVID-19 Outbreak in Asia and the Pacific: A Gender Lens.* New York.

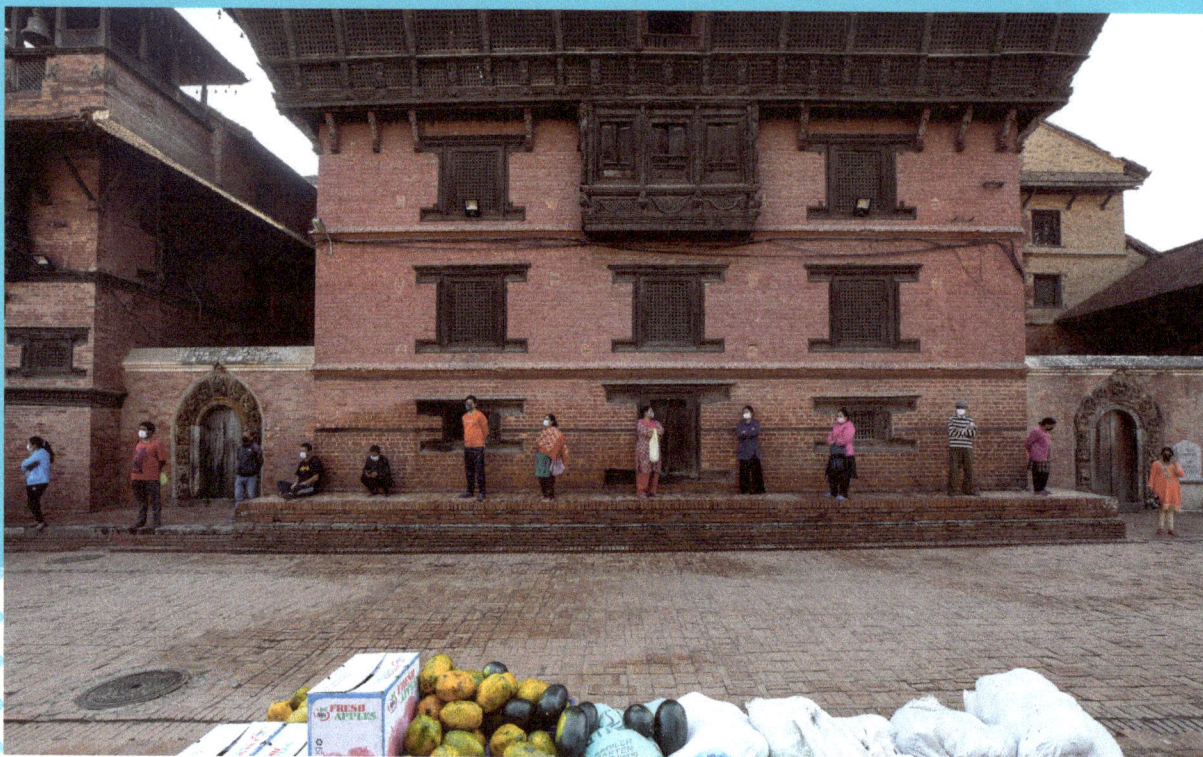

Disadvantaged and vulnerable. The crisis has worsened the situation of the urban poor as most live in unsafe and overcrowded areas.

3 Key Approaches for Cities During and After the Pandemic

Cities in DMCs can draw lessons from other cities around the world on how to implement more effective emergency responses and proactively plan their immediate actions. While pursuing such immediate actions to recover from the initial pandemic shocks, cities should not lose sight of short- and medium-term goals of enhancing safety, resilience, and livability. Cities can consider the following approaches:

(i) Cities experience varying impacts from COVID-19 and are not equal in their capacity to respond to crisis. Therefore, while learning from others and in planning their response, they should consider socioeconomic and political factors, such as but not limited to demographic profile and population characteristics; economic capabilities and income levels; geographic features; urban infrastructure and pre-COVID-19 service standards; and regulatory frameworks, devolution of powers, available resources, and personnel requirements.

(ii) Cities are making a wide range of decisions that can impact immediate prevention and protection measures (e.g., testing and tracking of COVID-19 cases, distributing food and subsistence allowances to the most vulnerable people) and longer-term paths to recovery.

(iii) A long-term approach should be factored into the immediate response as much as possible to achieve more strategic goals and objectives that will enable cities to "build back better."

(iv) COVID-19 provides a unique opportunity for cities to upscale innovation and use online tools and digital solutions through proven and new technologies, such as Internet of Things-based systems; artificial intelligence (e.g., for contact tracing and identifying potential COVID-19 cases); blockchain (e.g., for more secure communications and transactions); mobile applications (e.g., for citizens' awareness and education); teleworking (e.g., for work-from-home arrangements, distance learning, and skills development);[4] and network management technologies (e.g., for operation of municipal infrastructure utilities, networks, and services).

(v) Cities should continue to work in an inclusive manner to plan and prioritize their immediate actions to address the needs and take into account the potential abilities of the most vulnerable people (e.g., low-income residents, slum residents, informal sector workers, migrant workers, pavement dwellers, homeless people, single-parent households, the elderly, women and children, persons with disabilities, minorities, and migrants). Local governments can adopt differentiated approaches for such groups to support them in complying with prescribed public health and safety measures.

(vi) Cities, in consultation with the private sector and the civil society, need to carefully balance the health and well-being of their citizens. Both the drivers for local economic development and the specific capabilities possible under the constrained quarantine conditions and restrictions should be considered in identifying livelihood opportunities.

(vii) Cities need to work with national governments to ensure effective implementation of nationwide (or statewide, as appropriate) measures (e.g., quarantine directions, fiscal stimulus packages for workers and MSMEs, special social protection measures) or develop location-specific responses in line with national frameworks and initiatives.[5]

---

[4] M. Haag 2020. Manhattan Faces a Reckoning if Working from Home Becomes the Norm. *The New York Times*. 13 May.

[5] Organisation for Economic Co-operation and Development (OECD). 2020. Tackling Coronavirus (COVID-19) Contributing to a Global Effort: Cities Policy Responses. Paris.

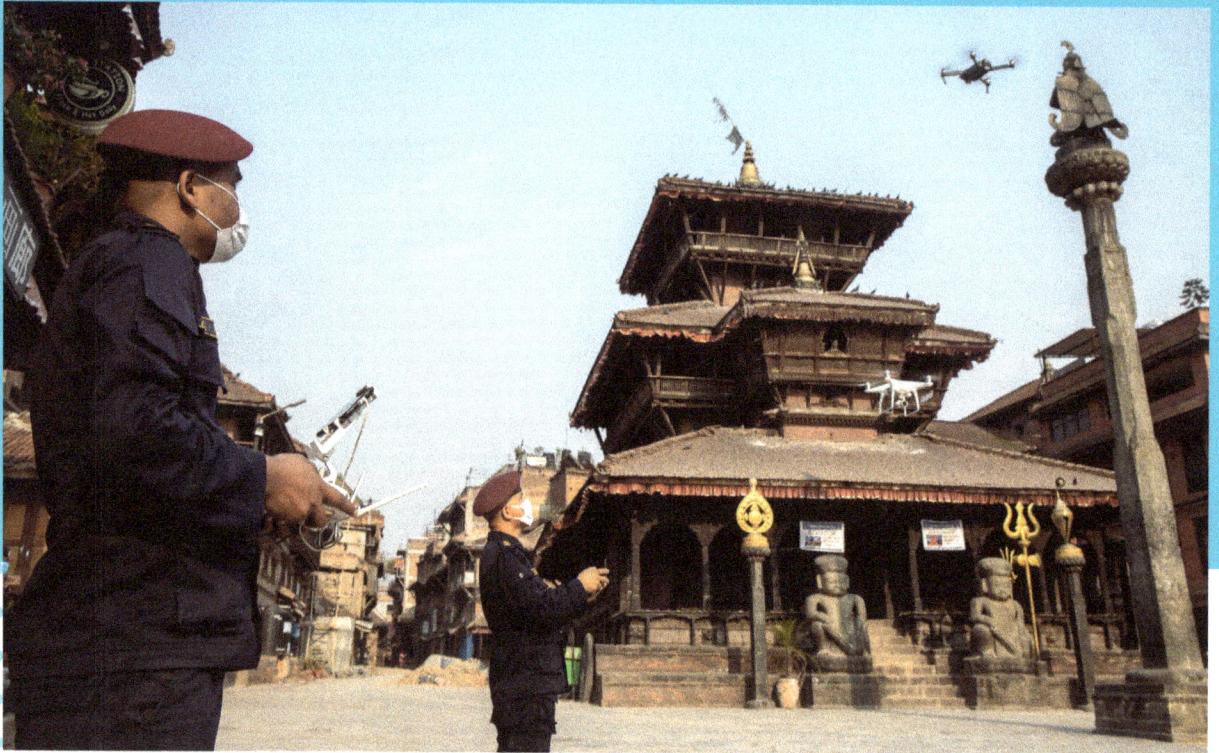

Innovating to combat COVID-19. Nepalese Police uses a drone to monitor lockdown in Bhaktapur district, Nepal.

4 Post-COVID-19 Emergency Response and Immediate Actions for Livable Cities

Adapting to the crisis to sustain urban services. Sustaining and improving the provision of and access to urban infrastructure and services are essential to tackling the risks posed by any pandemic. More than ever, effective services and quality infrastructure are required in cities, especially in slums and informal settlements, and for the poor and vulnerable communities. The issues and areas of intervention for emergency response and immediate actions are in line with OP4's three major outcomes (Figure 1). The specific actions that cities should consider implementing are summarized in Table 1.

Figure 1: Making Cities More Livable—Post-COVID-19 Emergency Response and Immediate Actions

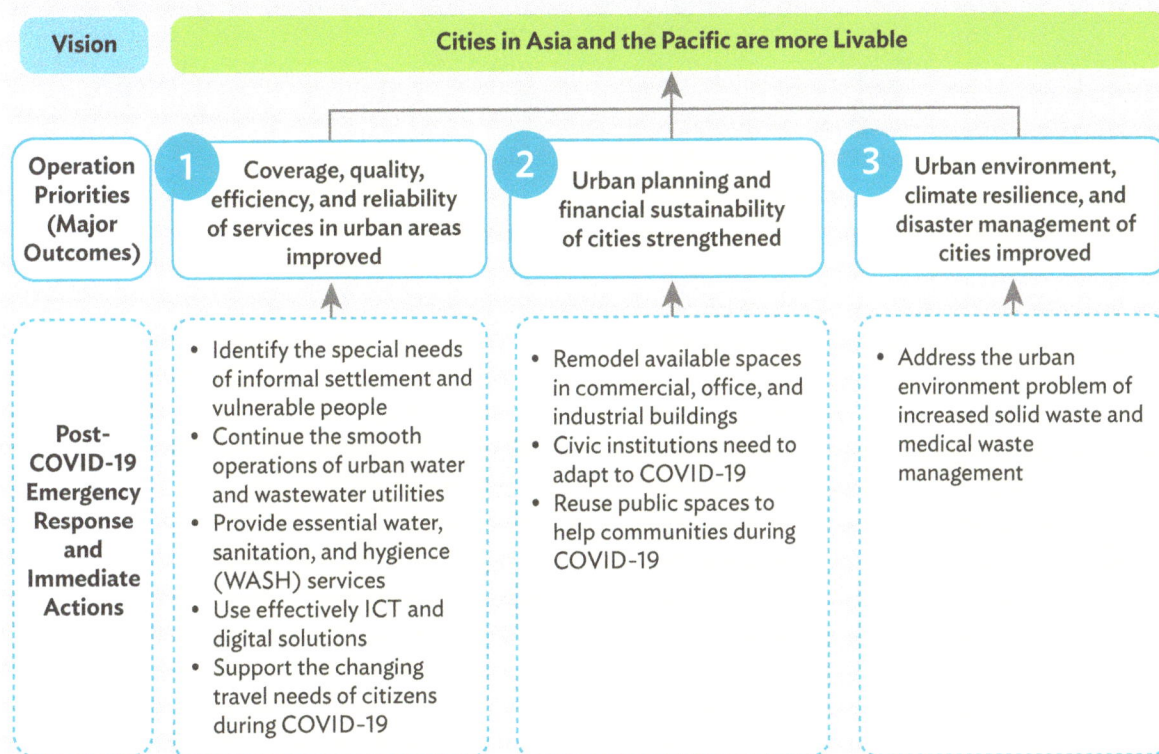

Vision	Cities in Asia and the Pacific are more Livable

Operation Priorities (Major Outcomes)	**1** Coverage, quality, efficiency, and reliability of services in urban areas improved	**2** Urban planning and financial sustainability of cities strengthened	**3** Urban environment, climate resilience, and disaster management of cities improved
Post-COVID-19 Emergency Response and Immediate Actions	• Identify the special needs of informal settlement and vulnerable people • Continue the smooth operations of urban water and wastewater utilities • Provide essential water, sanitation, and hygiene (WASH) services • Use effectively ICT and digital solutions • Support the changing travel needs of citizens during COVID-19	• Remodel available spaces in commercial, office, and industrial buildings • Civic institutions need to adapt to COVID-19 • Reuse public spaces to help communities during COVID-19	• Address the urban environment problem of increased solid waste and medical waste management

ICT = information and communication technology.
Source: Asian Development Bank.

Table 1: Emergency Response and Immediate Actions Required for Livable Cities

Issues and Areas of Intervention	Actions to Be Taken
Livable Cities Pillar 1: Coverage, quality, efficiency, and reliability of services in urban areas improved	
Special needs of informal settlements and vulnerable people Since a one-size-fits-all approach is not recommended for cities, similar omnibus measures for all informal settlements are not effective. Measures and policies (e.g., resource provision, communication strategy, training, and support) need to be adapted based on the characteristics of the groups of vulnerable people and informal settlement, such as physical environment, climate, population size, cultural and linguistic factors, crime rates, and relationship with the state.	• Consult with people in informal settlements, community leaders, nongovernment organizations, and urban poor networks to identify the vulnerable people (e.g., slum residents, pavement dwellers, squatters, homeless persons, informal sector workers, and migrant workers) and collaborate on developing and implementing response plans. • Calculate overcrowding of informal settlements to account for physical distancing. • Develop an appropriate communication strategy and implementation mechanism, allocate resources, and monitor for effective results. • Customize communication messages to different target groups in informal settlements to stimulate the required behavioral changes. • Operationalize a temporary coronavirus disease (COVID-19) information center in each community to disseminate messages, illustrate and remind people of preventive tips, and assess the availability of core urban services along with health checkups.

continued on next page

Table 1 *continued*

Issues and Areas of Intervention	Actions to Be Taken
	• Take measures to continuously monitor the health and nutrition status and access to basic services of communities (e.g., nutrition status of mothers, infants, and children who are likely to be most affected due to supply chain disruptions) using technology and digital solutions, particularly for areas with high infection rates, for quick response and recovery.
Continued smooth operations of urban water and wastewater utilities Water and wastewater utilities need to provide uninterrupted and quality services during the pandemic and ensure a safe and healthy environment for all residents.	• Adopt and provide solutions in real-time and in a dynamic fashion to address evolving issues and challenges (e.g., in terms of significantly different demands across different parts of the networks in contrast to normal usage). • Conduct regular analysis of virus RNA concentrations in sewage samples to establish early warning systems for tracking the spread of COVID-19 in the catchment communities.[a] • Communicate regularly and effectively with customers to provide assurance, get feedback, and make appropriate changes (e.g., disruptions or resumption of services). • Focus on human resource plans with possible incentives to motivate and inspire the workforce, who are also considered as frontline workers providing essential services. • Provide adequate personal protective equipment (PPE) for the workers. • Continue regular utility operations and implement scheduled asset management plans of treatment plants, pumping stations, valves, meters, distribution networks, nonrevenue water (NRW), and billing and collection systems. • Maintain operational efficiency—despite reduced workforce and decreased on-site visits—with innovative methods and use of technologies for sustained investigations of leakages, reduction of NRW, and clearance of repair backlogs. • Consider temporary suspension of non-essential expansion works and home call outs. • Learn from the experiences of utilities with centralized control, command centers, and supervisory control and data acquisition (SCADA) systems that are more effective in tackling the disruption of services.
Provision of essential water, sanitation, and hygiene (WASH) services WASH is central to preventing the spread of COVID-19 and other diseases. Handwashing with water and soap kills the virus but requires the provision of uninterrupted water in sufficient quantities. It is also critical to have effective sanitation and proper hygiene for all the people in pandemic-affected areas.	• Establish and operationalize proper government structures (e.g., interministerial committees) to coordinate and monitor response to COVID-19 with due focus on WASH. • Remove cost barriers to water access and ensure adequate water for WASH. • Extend financial and technical support to service providers in implementing the necessary measures for WASH (i.e., provide financial support to water utilities, engage public and private water service providers to include low-coverage areas, exempt from taxes WASH-related products imported into the country, and open credit lines to WASH-related enterprises to help them survive). • Implement targeted measures for vulnerable people given their high exposure and vulnerability to COVID-19.[b]

continued on next page

Table 1 *continued*

Issues and Areas of Intervention	Actions to Be Taken
Need for effective use of information and communication technology and digital solutions Cities should use ICT and digital solutions to respond to urgent needs and demands of their respective communities. They can use available technologies and solutions and quickly adapt their own systems considering the local context to enable more informed decision-making. Such an approach would also support external coherence and harmonization of processes and workflows.	• Create and lead an organized system of coordination, data management, and research on the impacts of COVID-19 on urban populations. • Establish a mechanism for sharing relevant findings and key recommendations within national coordination structures to inform and adjust the multisector local and national response (e.g., online tax and tariff management system, online administrative approvals, and grievance redress system). • Support the national approach of local data management systems and platforms, considering affordability and reliability, along with the national statistical offices and data teams from the relevant ministries (e.g., health, transport, education, technology, national development, and trade) that oversee case management statistics. • Produce city-level tracking system for levels of preparedness and response to COVID-19.[c] • Coordinate with national and local governments to support solutions for consistent urban services during periods of restricted movement (e.g., movement of essential logistics, scale and location of necessary health-care facilities, required specific region and period of community quarantine, planning of public transport considering flexible working hours, online or mobile communication with residents to ensure timely information and minimize physical contact).
Support for the changing travel needs of citizens during COVID-19 Transport during the COVID-19 crisis has resulted in significant changes since travel demand focuses more on essential travels, while spaces are constrained due to the physical distancing requirement.	• Reallocate space to allow for more physically spaced out non-motorized and low-carbon modes of transport (e.g., walking and cycling) or for resilience-enhancing services (e.g., health care, food, and other essential services). • Explore and strengthen measures to manage excess post-quarantine personal car traffic. • Relax administrative rules regarding emergency light individual transport lanes and consider incentive schemes on shared micro-mobility. • Prioritize logistics in road and rail transport to ensure continued supply of essential goods. • Keep public mass transit open for essential workers' mobility considering physical distancing measures. • Provide funding for the deployment of more light individual transport lanes.

continued on next page

Table 1 *continued*

Issues and Areas of Intervention	Actions to Be Taken
Livable Cities Pillar 2: Urban planning and financial sustainability of cities strengthened	
Need to remodel available spaces in commercial, office, and industrial buildings These spaces need to adjust or limit gatherings and commercial activities, except for essential activities such as in supermarkets, pharmacies, banks, insurance, and postal services, which should apply stringent distancing measures before gradually shifting to overall confinement or vice versa.	• Recalculate the occupancy rate to account for social distancing and complement this with flexible work-time arrangements (e.g., considering the short- to medium-term plans regarding more staggered commuting, gathering patterns, and softened rush hour times). • Recalibrate building designs and systems to be more efficient, safe, and virus-free by establishing protocols for cleaning, maintenance, sanitization, and disinfection; auditing existing heating, ventilating, and air-conditioning systems; and maximizing outdoor air intake to increase the supply of fresh air.[d] Companies and building management can also use or install safety and protective features, such as infrared forehead thermometers, thermal scanners, disinfectant mats, protective covering, and wayfinding and information signs. • Review the legal and regulatory systems of building plan approvals to enhance, wherever possible, requirements for public health and social protection (e.g., housing, health care, open spaces, education, amenities). • Review plans of buildings scheduled for construction, demolition, renovation, or reconstruction in the light of new systems.
Civic institutions need to adapt to COVID-19 Similar to commercial spaces, civic institutions pose a high risk for COVID-19 transmission due to the concentration of people in such places. Complying with social distancing is critical in these areas to address COVID-19.	• Identify non-essential facilities to be closed. • Prepare protocols for entry and exit and designate the number of people allowed during meetings and activities for core civic institutions (e.g., places of worship, museums, concert halls or cultural centers, community centers) to follow the physical distance and safety requirements. • Consider changing operating hours to stretch out activities and avoid large volume of people. • Organize some activities online to allow regular access and programs to continue, especially for vulnerable people who may only have these services as their sole option (free) for religious, education, or cultural activities (e.g., prayer or masses, workshops or classes, theatrical performances, art exhibitions).
Reuse of public spaces to help communities during COVID-19 Public spaces become valuable in enabling emergency response to dense populations in cities.	• Identify and classify public spaces (e.g., open spaces, parks, community centers, reserved sites, roads, government buildings) to be utilized for public health care (e.g., additional medical facilities for testing, treatment, and containment), communal activities (e.g., mobile markets, distribution centers, parks, sports and wellness areas), and for temporary housing and working spaces for daily functions during the quarantine period (e.g., community kitchens, housing for medical and repatriated workers). • Repurpose and restructure spaces for wet markets considering human infection by animal-borne diseases and expand outside spaces to enable social distancing.

continued on next page

Issues and Areas of Intervention	Actions to Be Taken
	• Consider pedestrians and cyclists as important stakeholders and allow wider-spaced walking and cycling paths within the existing infrastructure for a walkable and bike-friendly city. • Introduce temporary barriers and fences and entry and exit procedures to limit and organize the number of people present in certain public spaces (e.g., parks or playgrounds). • Through community engagement, develop and separate infrastructure and spaces for the provision of temporary or alternative public transport or logistics for daily needs (e.g., food) and critical items (e.g., health-care equipment).
Livable Cities Pillar 3: Urban environment, climate resilience, and disaster management of cities improved	
Need to address urban environment problem of increased solid waste and medical waste management The World Health Organization (WHO) advises that any system adopting best practices in infectious waste management can also manage the waste potentially infected with the virus causing COVID-19.[e] For medical waste management, it is recommended that all countries consider reviewing their infectious medical waste management system and refine their protocols as appropriate.	• Identify and implement the best collection, treatment, and management approaches according to the prevailing national system (e.g., considering both incineration and non-incineration methods, as appropriate). • Review existing national standards and systems and make quick amendments wherever appropriate. • Identify and monitor infectious waste, including medical waste, at source (e.g., from hospitals, laboratories, and quarantine facilities) and secure locations and availability of intermediate storage as much as possible and when safe to do so.[f] • Given the huge increase in infectious medical waste, arrange temporary storage (e.g., refrigerated shipping containers) with a suitably color-coded liner, and implement the usual collection and treatment systems. • Collect and transport the infectious waste in leakproof containers labeled with a biohazard symbol. • Send the waste for disposal or recycling after disinfection. Any infectious material that could potentially be reused should be destroyed or rendered unusable. • Consider strict entry, exit, and operation procedures at public recycling facilities to prevent overcrowding. • Collaborate with civil society organizations in the informal waste recycling sector to distribute face masks and other personal protective equipment to waste pickers.

[a] E. Stannard and J. Papp. 2020. Sewage Reveals COVID-19 Totals: New Haven Register. *Yale Global Online*. 28 May.
[b] Sanitation and Water for All. 2020. *Global Ministerial Webinar on Making WASH a Political and Financial Priority in the Time of COVID-19*. 9 April.
[c] UNICEF. 2020. *How COVID-19 is Changing the World: A Statistical Perspective*. New York.
[d] AECOM. 2020. *The Future of Workplace Re-occupancy*. Los Angeles, CA.
[e] Health Care Without Harm. 2020. *Health Care Waste Management: Coronavirus Update*. 24 March.
[f] ADB. 2020. *Managing Infectious Medical Waste During the COVID-19 Pandemic*. Manila.

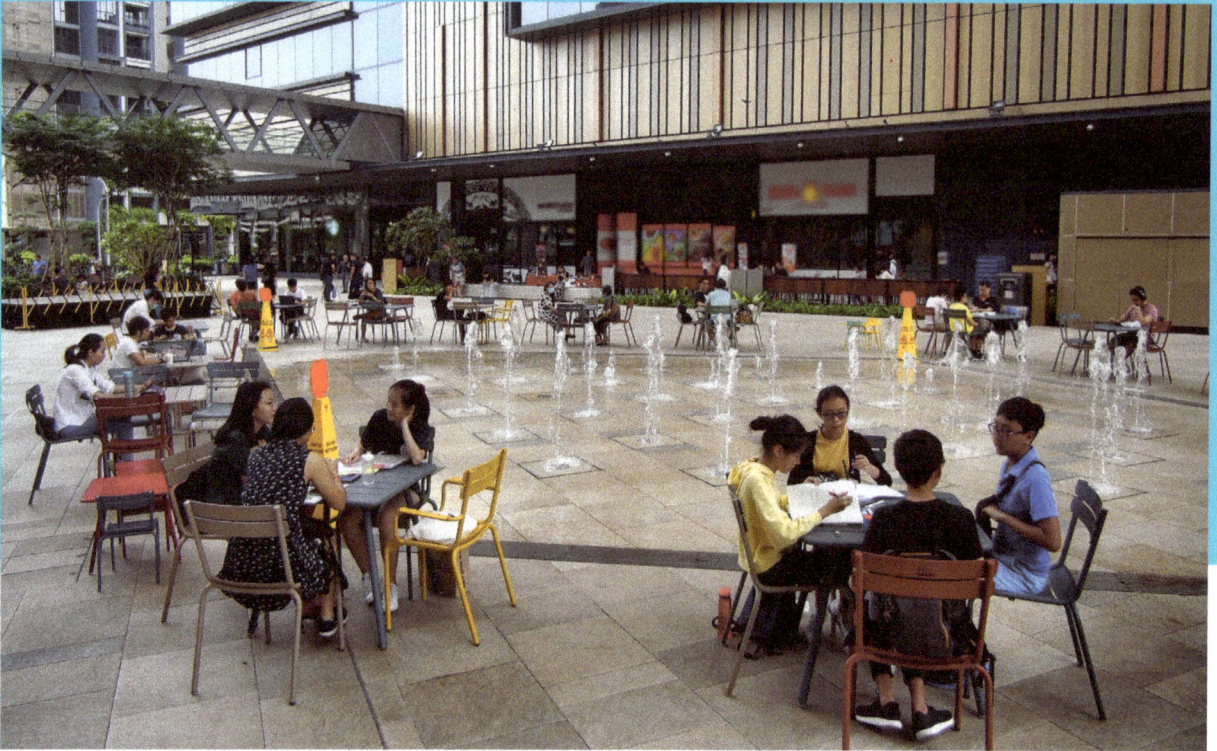

Social distancing is critical. Commercial establishments need to follow protocols to avoid the spread of the virus.

5 Build Back Better: Post-Pandemic Livable Cities

Redesign cities for resilience, inclusivity, and well-being. The COVID-19 pandemic exposes existing fault lines with respect to poor physical infrastructure, unequal access to core urban services, and suboptimal densities resulting in overcrowded cities. It is time to revisit the urban strategies and revise the urbanization process and practices to build back better post-pandemic cities. For example, there is a debate on what is the optimal density for cities in the wake of the pandemic— there is no straightforward answer. Cities with higher levels of access and quality of services and more public spaces can better handle greater densities. Higher densities with lower levels of access and quality of services and limited public spaces cause overcrowded localities in cities. On what is the optimum population density, each locality in a city needs to be examined carefully. Each city can use its specific context and right parameters to assess if it has a livable and healthy density in each of its localities (i.e., appropriate number of dwelling units and people, and adequate urban services per unit area in each locality of the city) or a risky overcrowding condition (e.g., excessive number of dwelling units and people, and inadequate urban services per unit area in each locality of the city).[6] Each city needs to consider its own context and the elements of livability (e.g., green, competitive, inclusive, and resilient city) and the focus areas (low-carbon development, climate resilience, energy efficiency city) while determining optimum density for each of its locality.

---

6   A. Dasgupta. 2020. *After the Crisis: How COVID-19 Can Drive Transformational Change in Cities. The City Fix.* 28 April; and R. van den Berg. 2020. *How Will COVID-19 Affect Urban Planning? The City Fix.* 10 April.

Cities are economic powerhouse and innovation hubs that can improve livelihoods and trigger prosperity. As cities work to mitigate the immediate crisis and plan about recovery, it is important that they prioritize investments that will build resilience and inclusivity in the short- and medium-term so that governments, households, and firms can weather future shocks and stresses, while increasing healthy urban lives.[7] To help cities become more healthy, environmentally sustainable, and resilient, urban infrastructure and development projects have to provide support on building resilience to disasters and climate change as well as to pandemics and diseases. Similarly, to accelerate economic recovery in an inclusive manner, cities should integrate labor markets with transport and economic sectors without losing sight of MSMEs and social protection for vulnerable people. Finally, cities should plan for spatial areas that have been particularly impacted by COVID-19 (e.g., public markets, business districts, public transport systems, health and waste facilities) and for vulnerable people who have been most adversely affected in the current crisis (e.g., low-income residents, slum residents, informal sector workers and migrant workers, pavement dwellers, homeless residents, single-parent households, the elderly, women and children, people with disabilities, minorities). Such projects should also reflect the lessons learned from the pandemic in terms of everyday and emergency uses of public spaces and infrastructure services, and the recommended design approaches, building standards, and flexibility to respond to changing conditions and needs.

Figure 2 shows how cities can adapt to the "new normal" in the short- and medium-term in line with OP4. Table 2 lays out the specific areas of interventions and actions for consideration.

Figure 2: Making Cities More Livable—Post-COVID-19 Short- and Medium-Term Actions for the New Normal

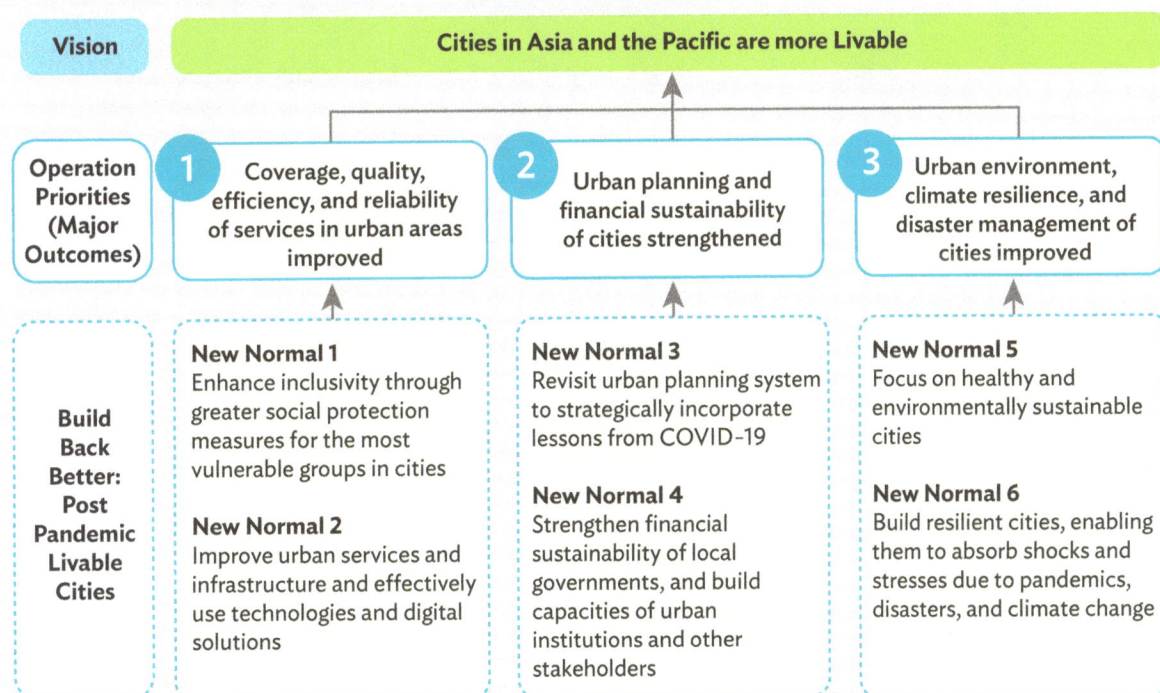

COVID-19 = coronavirus disease.

Source: Asian Development Bank.

The New Climate Economy. 2020. *NCE Key Message Pack—Special Edition on COVID-19.*

Table 2: Short- and Medium-Term Actions for Post-Pandemic Livable Cities

Areas of Intervention	Actions for Consideration
Livable Cities Pillar 1: Coverage, quality, efficiency, and reliability of services in urban areas improved	
Enhance inclusivity through greater social protection measures for the most vulnerable groups in cities	• Identify the special needs of different groups of vulnerable people (e.g., low-income residents, slum residents, informal sector workers and migrant workers, pavement dwellers, homeless residents, single-parent households, the elderly, women and children, people with disabilities, minorities), and prepare special programs focusing on social protection and economic needs of each group. • Provide adequate resources and devise implementation mechanisms to implement special programs for each vulnerable group (e.g., provision of affordable rental housing and legal protection measures against exploitation of informal sector workers and migrant workers, adequate urban services for slum residents). • Conduct regular census of people in vulnerable groups and establish digital social registers or data banks linked with their unique identification numbers (e.g., social security number or Aadhar number in India) and bank accounts for financial inclusion, and plan for implementation of fast and transparent direct benefit transfer schemes. • Promote economic activities, jobs, and entrepreneurships for eligible and willing vulnerable groups through special measures, as appropriate, such as support for project development and financing of investments and working capital, tax relief measures, lower development charges, and streamlined administrative processes. • Ensure that adequate and affordable core urban services (Table 3) are available to all vulnerable groups at the same standards available to the general population. • Reconsider the use of overcrowded public transport allowing medium-dense (not overcrowded) residential (re)development, including affordable housing for the vulnerable people in cities where economic activities exist.[a] • Reconsider the use of overcrowded public transport for redesigning multimodal integrated transport, giving priority to nonmotorized and low-carbon modes (e.g., walking and cycling). • Conduct research and develop prototypes and techniques for cost-effective projects for the vulnerable people.

continued on next page

Table 2 *continued*

Areas of Intervention	Actions for Consideration
Improve urban services and infrastructure and effectively use technologies and digital solutions	• Improve access to quality infrastructure and services (e.g., water supply, sanitation, power, transport, and social services) that are energy-efficient, pro-poor, gender-responsive, disabilities-inclusive, and sustainable while promoting a smart and digitized city. • Review, assess, and develop a comprehensive policy and regulatory framework on data governance, including data acquisition, processing, sharing, and ownership. • Identify and support innovative ideas for urban improvement and new smart city solutions through incubator labs, knowledge hubs, and hackathons that, among others, engage citizens and the private sector. • Consider government budgets as well as financial support from private sector financing for smart city initiatives (e.g., PPP for funding, technical expertise, and innovation). • Attract and upskill digital capacities through knowledge sharing between cities (e.g., twinning arrangements with more developed cities, partnerships with technology providers, academia, or NGOs). • Implement a program management unit with sufficient capacity for planning, coordination, and implementation of a smart city initiative.[b] • Integrate hard and soft digital infrastructures in urban planning and development to improve urban services (e.g., early monitoring system for disaster and disease, medical consultation, remote supervision by utilizing SCADA, decentralized one-stop-shop service facilities, and leveraging the mobile big data). • Promote citizens' active engagement and empowerment but also respecting individual privacy, and strengthen data security to address citizens' concerns on surveillance.
Livable Cities Pillar 2: Urban planning and financial sustainability of cities strengthened	
Revisit urban planning systems to strategically incorporate lessons from COVID-19	• Coordinate with relevant authorities such as for transport, health, land resources, building and construction, energy, environment, water, park and public spaces, food, civil aviation, maritime and port, tourism, and labor and workplace to provide a solid baseline for the response and contingency plan (e.g., mainstream the additional precautions and safety standards to address the pandemic), so as to consider appropriate new government arrangements across different levels of governance. • Analyze the existing and planned population changes, demographic profiles, and economic capability of the cities considering the revised post-COVID-19 standards to determine the optimum urban density without overcrowding urban spaces and overburdening urban infrastructure. • Coordinate with national and provincial governments for balanced regional development, focusing on developing small and medium cities as alternate economic hubs to megacities and metropolitan areas (e.g., shifting economic activities in manufacturing and services to the prioritized secondary cities or making secondary cities attractive for informal sector workers and migrant workers from the rural areas).

continued on next page

Table 2 *continued*

Areas of Intervention	Actions for Consideration
	• Reidentify the required open and natural areas to provide healthy spaces for inhabitants' physical activities in the long run (e.g., urban sponge absorbing air pollution to improve urban environment quality and potential areas for response, such as shelter, temporary services, or supply delivery).[c] • Promote collaboration with governments and the private sector for efficient and innovative real estate and infrastructure projects (e.g., urban regeneration of business district or transit-oriented development through PPP, land-based financing, and land-pooling system) for sustainable urban growth.
Strengthen the financial sustainability of local governments, and build the capacities of urban institutions and other stakeholders	• Considering the impacts of the pandemic, develop a strategy to strengthen financial sustainability of local governments through maximizing revenue (e.g., taxes, tariffs, and intergovernment transfers); developing more robust data-based collection system; catalyzing additional revenue sources (e.g., private sector participation, PPPs, bonds, guarantees, municipal development funds and pooled financing, enhancing creditworthiness to raise capital on markets, and using infrastructure as an asset class); and rationalizing expenditures (e.g., improving efficiencies, cutting nonessential costs).[d] • Work closely with the national government in creating or strengthening institutions such as financial intermediaries to support local authorities in preparing, appraising, and implementing projects for urban and social infrastructure. • Review existing urban institutions in cities by considering their responses to COVID-19 and develop capacity-building plans including revised organizational structure, if required, for each urban institution. • Learn and apply relevant lessons from cities that were successful during the COVID-19 crisis and other such disasters and pandemics in terms of institutional capacities; service delivery and stakeholder engagement; internal governance systems, processes, and documentation; human capital development and skills-building systems; project management, sustainable operation, and management of assets; and use of technologies and digital solutions. • Provide adequate resources and design implementation and monitoring mechanisms to effectively execute capacity-building programs. • Ensure transparent and consistent coordination and coherence across different levels of governance. • Promote collaboration with external stakeholders such as other cities, academic institutions, and private development partners. • Establish partnerships with community-based groups and leaders to build capacities of communities and citizens, improve service delivery to citizens, and complement top–down decision-making. • Promote knowledge generation and innovation, especially localized approaches to urban development from local communities.

continued on next page

Table 2 *continued*

Areas of Intervention	Actions for Consideration
Livable Cities Pillar 3: Urban environment, climate resilience, and disaster management of cities improved	
Focus on healthy and environmentally sustainable cities	• Develop locally relevant principles for a healthy and environmentally sustainable city (e.g., physical distancing in urban space, public health system and standard, adjustment of public transport operations, health impact assessments, and healthy and age-friendly city action and management planning for a pandemic and economically disruptive events) (footnote a). • Practice systemic thinking on healthy and environmentally sustainable city and mainstream these principles in all aspects of urban governance—urban planning and design, infrastructure projects, cross-sector and cross-jurisdictional municipal functions, capacity-building activities, operations of urban services, and engagement with citizens and other stakeholders. • Promote energy efficiency using renewable energy to reduce demand for energy and environment impacts and increase access to heating and cooling system for the vulnerable groups in cities. • Review risk-sensitive land use management (e.g., change of land use), nature-based solution, circular economy practices, and low-carbon transformation to encourage flexible and mixed-use (re)development for healthy and environmentally sustainable programs and facilities.
Build resilient cities, enabling them to absorb shocks and stresses due to pandemics, disasters, and climate change	• Develop locally relevant principles for cities to be resilient to disasters, climate change, and economically disruptive events (e.g., safe workplace principles, contingency plan for community quarantine). • Practice systemic thinking on safe and resilient cities and mainstream these principles in all aspects of urban governance—urban planning and design, infrastructure projects, cross-sector and cross-jurisdictional municipal functions, capacity-building activities, operations of urban services, and engagement with citizens and other stakeholders. • Promote climate-resilient delivery of core urban service standards (Table 3). • Plan for disaster preparedness and emergency response, including effective forecasting, early warning systems, and proper communication and consultation strategies; and provide adequate resources for implementing such plans. • Utilize publicly owned land or revitalize obsolete or abandoned facilities (e.g., redevelopment of inefficient infrastructure and unsafe and dilapidated buildings) for resilient spaces and infrastructures.

NGO = nongovernment organization, PPP = public–private partnership, SCADA = supervisory control and data acquisition.
[a] ADB. 2020. *Working Paper Series on Healthy and Age-friendly Cities in the PRC*. Manila.
[b] ADB. 2020. *Smart City Pathways for Developing Asia: An Analytical Framework and Guidance*. Manila.
[c] A. Pérez. 2020. Urban Planning in Times of COVID-19—Resilience and Inclusiveness. *Heriland*. 3 April.
[d] ADB. 2020. *Financial Sustainability of Cities*. Manila.
Source: Asian Development Bank.

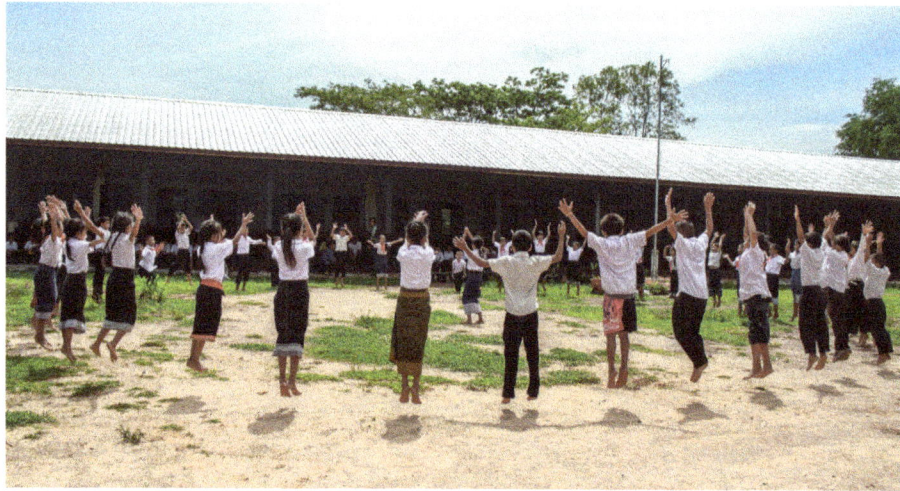

Education for all. Core urban service standards include ensuring access of inhabitants to compulsory education and training.

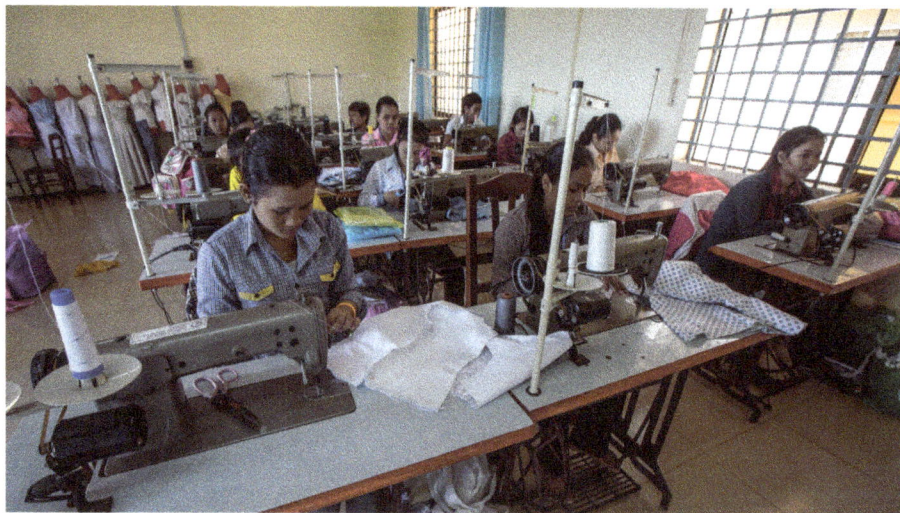

Decent work. Investing into the local economy and creating jobs are important elements of urban service standards.

Required Core Urban Service Standards

Core urban service standards will help in planning and building the required urban and social infrastructure facilities (Table 3). Such standards will also ensure access to adequate, safe, and affordable housing and basic services. These will also support pro-poor and inclusive cities with a healthy urban environment, as well as resilient cities through the strengthened disaster preparedness and emergency response facilities. The detailed and required standards should consider the nationwide status of urbanization, population, economic development, finance, capacities of implementation, operation and management, applicable regulation and policy, and existing relationship and possible coordination among various tiers of governments. As these could be long-term ambitions with substantial budget requirements for some cities, it is important to undertake prioritized planning for the most optimal interventions (e.g., urban [re] development and infrastructure with innovative financial and regulatory supports) so that the proposed new norms could be achieved gradually and efficiently.

Table 3: Required Core Urban Service Standards

Element		Required Core Urban Service Standards
Public health/ welfare	Primary health-care services (clinic)/medical services (hospital)	• Primary health care service within certain time and/or distance • Primary health care service provision within certain square meter (m^2), vehicles, beds, and/or officers per capita
	Emergency services	• Medical and firefighting treatment service by appropriate equipment within certain time (and/or distance) • Emergency response service provision within certain m^2/vehicles/beds/officers per capita
	Water, sanitation, and hygiene (WASH)	• Distribution rate per capita (or household)
	Care for vulnerable groups	• Average area (m^2) of care service for each vulnerable group (youth, children, women, elderly, persons with disabilities)
Education	Nursery/elementary school/ middle school/high school/ college	• Participation in compulsory education including home learning (% of age cohort)
	Continuing education and training	• Average area (m^2) per capita (across all age categories)
Urban services/ urban infrastructure/ social infrastructure	Affordable housing	• Ratio of affordable housing to total number of housing • Access (%) of total urban population (or household)
	Water supply	• Water supply to consumers (duration, pressure, and quality of water)
	Wastewater management	• Proportion (%) of wastewater collection and treatment • Solid waste collected (%) and treated (%)
	Solid waste management/ medical waste management	• Medical waste collected (%) and treated (%) • Capacity of appropriate treatment facility (in remaining years and/or million cubic meters)
	Heating/cooling	• Distribution rate per capita (or household)
	Public transport	• Modal share between rail, bus, other public transport, individual car, motorcycle, cycling, and walking • Affordability and frequency (accessibility) • Available parking space per residential unit or business area
	Electricity	• Affordability, accessibility, and stability
	Internet	• Distribution rate per capita (or household) and the stability and speed of internet
Economic activity	Job training/ MSMEs consulting/ local investment/ job creation	• Number of entrepreneurs and MSMEs advised/supported through local business centers/programs • Growth of small business registrations • Availability of the number of job trainings and MSMEs consulting • Investments into local economy (year-on-year development in local currency, inflation-adjusted) • Number of jobs created (year-on-year % change, and absolute figure)

continued on next page

Table 3 *continued*

Element		Required Core Urban Service Standards
Culture/leisure/ community	Community facilities cultural facilities/ sports facilities/ libraries	• Average area (m²) per capita
	Public plazas/ public parks/ playgrounds	• Average area (m²) per capita
	Corner shops/markets	• Average area (m²) per capita • Proximity of public areas in time or distance per neighborhood
Safety	Police facilities	• Number of police officers per capita
	Firefighting facilities	• Number of firefighting officers per capita
	Disaster emergency facilities	• Average area (m²) of disaster prevention facilities (e.g., for earthquake, flood, landslide) per capita (or household)

MSMEs = micro, small, and medium-sized enterprises.
Source: Asian Development Bank.

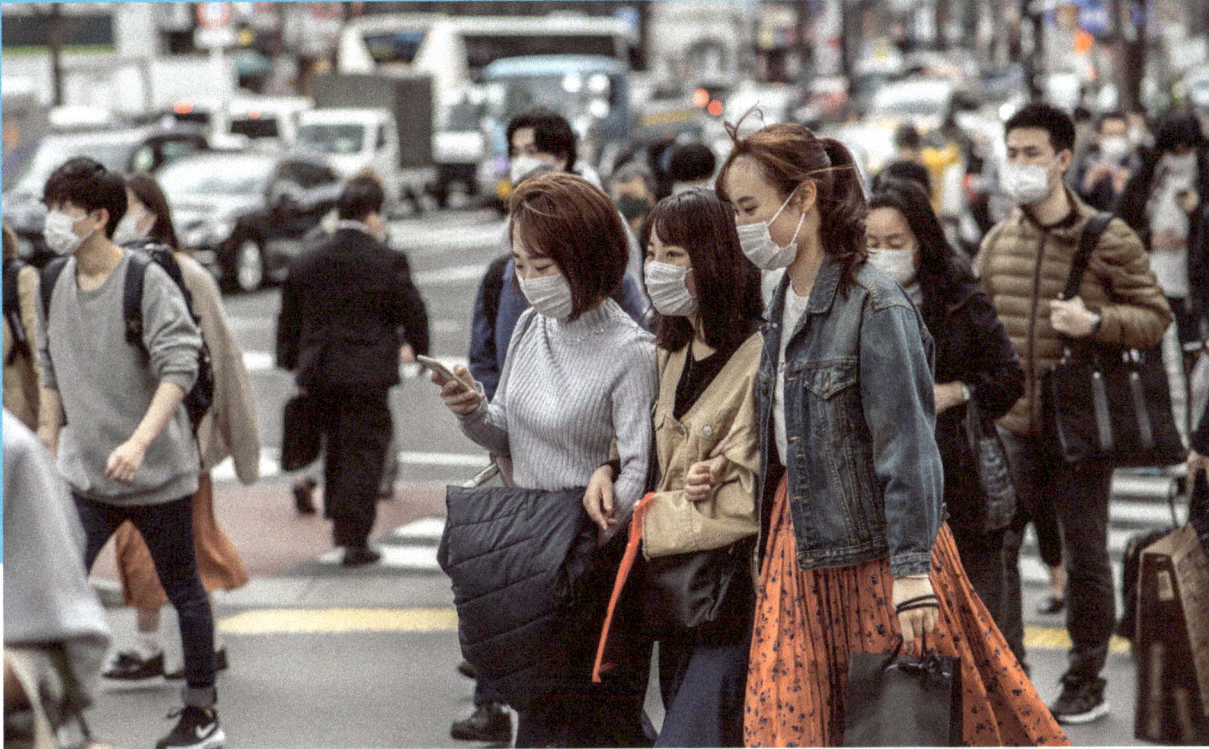

Building back better. ADB commits to continue working with its member countries to make cities in Asia and the Pacific more healthy, resilient, and inclusive.

(6) Potential ADB Support and Way Forward

Aligning ADB's Urban Sector Portfolio to Address COVID-19 Impacts on DMCs

The average project commitments in ADB's urban sector are about $2 billion per year, and are expected to be the same amount in 2020. To address the impacts of COVID-19, ADB's livable cities projects will be designed to help cities in DMCs become more healthy, inclusive, and resilient, and support local economic development and creation of well-paying jobs for the citizens. Specifically, livable cities projects will include components to support, among others, the following: (i) integrated urban planning process and coordination across departments and local administrative boundaries to strategically incorporate lessons from COVID-19 for safe and healthy cities; (ii) greater social protection measures, including affordable housing with integrated urban services, for the most vulnerable groups in cities; and (iii) improvement of urban environments, focusing on uninterrupted utility operations, WASH, wastewater and fecal sludge management, and solid waste and medical waste management. The livable cities projects will also strengthen financial sustainability; support financial inclusion; improve urban services through the use of technologies and digital solutions; and build capacities of urban institutions, communities, and other stakeholders.

Way Forward for Post-Pandemic Cities

Most cities in DMCs are currently focusing their resources on the immediate management and response to COVID-19. While this is critical, cities paying attention to how immediate actions align with the short- and medium-term measures will gain an advantage toward building back better. It will also be useful to understand how short- and medium-term actions synergize with other ongoing or planned investments and broader agendas (e.g., national development strategies, public investment plans, ADB's Strategy 2030, the Sustainable Development Goals and Agenda 2030, and nationally determined contributions in line with the Paris Climate Agreement). While not discounting the human toll and tragedy of the pandemic, this crisis can be turned into an opportunity and momentum to reduce inequalities of access and make cities more safe, healthy, environmentally sustainable, resilient, and inclusive in a post-COVID-19 world. ADB will also help cities understand their challenges and opportunities as they prepare their own visions, plans, and road maps; take appropriate actions to address pandemics; and implement projects to create more livable cities.

References

ADB. 2019. *Strategy 2030 Operational Plan for Priority 4: Making Cities More Livable, 2019–2024.* Manila.

————. 2020. *Managing Infectious Medical Waste during the COVID-19 Pandemic.* Manila.

————. 2020. *Smart City Pathways for Developing Asia: An Analytical Framework and Guidance.* Manila.

————. 2020. *Working Paper Series on Healthy and Age-friendly Cities in the PRC.* Manila.

————. 2021. Contemporary Issues for Creating Livable Asian Cities. Unpublished.

A. Dasgupta. 2020. *After the Crisis: How COVID-19 Can Drive Transformational Change in Cities. The City Fix.* 28 April.

AECOM. 2020. *The Future of Workplace Re-occupancy.* Los Angeles, CA.

A. Pérez. 2020. Urban Planning in Times of COVID-19—Resilience and Inclusiveness. *Heriland.* 3 April.

E. Stannard and J. Papp. 2020. Sewage Reveals COVID-19 Totals: New Haven Register. *Yale Global Online.* 28 May.

Health Care Without Harm. 2020. *Health Care Waste Management: Coronavirus Update.* 24 March.

M. Haag 2020. *Manhattan Faces a Reckoning if Working from Home Becomes the Norm. The New York Times.* 13 May.

Organisation for Economic Co-operation and Development (OECD). 2020. *Tackling Coronavirus (COVID-19) Contributing to a Global Effort: Cities Policy Responses.* Paris.

R. van den Berg. 2020. *How Will COVID-19 Affect Urban Planning? The City Fix.* 10 April.

Sanitation and Water for All. 2020. *Global Ministerial Webinar on Making WASH a Political and Financial Priority in the Time of COVID-19.* 9 April.

Stannard. E and J. Papp. 2020. Sewage Reveals COVID-19 Totals: New Haven Register. *Yale Global Online.* 28 May.

The New Climate Economy. 2020. *NCE Key Message Pack—Special Edition on COVID-19.*

United Nations Economic and Social Commission for Asia and the Pacific (UNESCAP). 2019. *The Future of Asian and Pacific Cities.* Bangkok.

United Nations Children's Fund (UNICEF). 2020. *How COVID-19 is Changing the World: A Statistical Perspective.*

UN Women. 2020. *The First 100 Days of the COVID-19 Outbreak in Asia and the Pacific: A Gender Lens.* New York.

www.ingramcontent.com/pod-product-compliance
Lightning Source LLC
Chambersburg PA
CBHW041122280326

41928CB00061B/3497